MedicalCenter.com

The Key Facts
On Cancer Types

The Key Facts on Cancer: Volume II

Everything You Need to Know About Cancer Types

-Usable Medical Information for the Patient-

By Patrick W. Nee

www.MedicalCenter.com

Published by:

MedicalCenter.com

96 Walter Street/ Suite 200

Boston, MA 02131, USA

Tel: 617-354-7722

www.MedicalCenter.com

manager@medicalcenter.com

The Key Facts on Cancer Series

Volume I: The Key Facts on Cancer Treatment

Volume II: The Key Facts on Cancer Types

Volume III: The Key Facts on Cancer Risk Factors and Causes

Volume IV: The Key Facts on Cancer Prevention

Volume V: The Key Facts on Cancer Detection and Diagnosis

Volume VI: The Key Facts on Coping With Cancer & Cancer Resources

Table of Contents

Chapter 1: Introduction

What is Cancer?

Cancer is a term used for diseases in which abnormal cells divide without control and are able to invade other tissues. Cancer cells can spread to other parts of the body through the blood and lymph systems.

Cancer is not just one disease but many diseases. There are more than 100 different types of cancer. Most cancers are named for the organ or type of cell in which they start - for example, cancer that begins in the colon is called colon cancer; cancer that begins in melanocytes of the skin is called melanoma.

Cancer types can be grouped into broader categories. The main categories of cancer include:

- **Carcinoma**- cancer that begins in the skin or in tissues that line or cover internal organs. There are a number of subtypes of carcinoma, including adenocarcinoma, basal cell carcinoma,squamous cell carcinoma, and transitional cell carcinoma.
- **Sarcoma** - cancer that begins in bone, cartilage, fat, muscle, blood vessels, or other connective or supportive tissue.

- *Leukemia* - cancer that starts in blood-forming tissue such as the bone marrow and causes large numbers of abnormal blood cells to be produced and enter the blood.
- *Lymphoma and myeloma* - cancers that begin in the cells of the immune system.
- *Central nervous system cancers* - cancers that begin in the tissues of the brain and spinal cord.

Origins of Cancer

All cancers begin in cells, the body's basic unit of life. To understand cancer, it's helpful to know what happens when normal cells become cancer cells.

The body is made up of many types of cells. These cells grow and divide in a controlled way to produce more cells as they are needed to keep the body healthy. When cells become old or damaged, they die and are replaced with new cells. However, sometimes this orderly process goes wrong. The genetic material (DNA) of a cell can become damaged or changed, producing mutations that affect normal cell growth and division. When this happens, cells do not die when they should and new cells form when the body does not need them. The extra cells may form a mass of tissue called a tumor.

Not all tumors are cancerous; tumors can be benign or malignant.

- **Benign tumors** aren't cancerous. They can often be removed, and, in most cases, they do not come back. Cells in benign tumors do not spread to other parts of the body.
- **Malignant tumors** are cancerous. Cells in these tumors can invade nearby tissues and spread to other parts of the body. The spread of cancer from one part of the body to another is called metastasis.

Some cancers do not form tumors. For example, leukemia is a cancer of the bone marrow and blood.

Cancer Statistics

A report from the nation's leading cancer organizations shows that rates of death in the United States from all cancers for men and women continued to fall between 2005 and 2009, the most recent reporting period available.

Estimated new cases and deaths from cancer in the United States in 2013:

- *New cases*: 1,660,290 (does not include nonmelanoma skin cancers)
- *Deaths*: 580,350

The risk of developing many types of cancer can be reduced by practicing healthy lifestyle habits, such as eating a healthy diet, getting regular exercise, and not smoking. Also, the sooner a cancer is found and treatment begins, the better the chances are that the treatment will be successful.

Chapter 2: Bone Cancer

- Cancer that starts in the bone is uncommon.
- Pain is the most common symptom of bone cancer.
- Surgery is the usual treatment for bone cancer.
- With modern surgical techniques, 9 out of 10 people who have bone cancer in an arm or leg may not need amputation.
- Because bone cancer can come back after treatment, regular follow-up visits are important.
- People with bone cancer are encouraged to enroll in clinical trials (research studies) that explore new treatments.

What is bone cancer?

Bone cancer is a malignant (cancerous) tumor of the bone that destroys normal bone tissue. Not all bone tumors are malignant. In fact, benign (noncancerous) bone tumors are more common than malignant ones. Both malignant and benign bone tumors may grow and compress healthy bone tissue, but benign tumors do not spread, do not destroy bone tissue, and are rarely a threat to life.

Malignant tumors that begin in bone tissue are called primary bone cancer. Cancer that metastasizes (spreads) to the bones from other parts of the body, such as the breast, lung, or prostate, is called metastatic cancer, and is named for the organ or tissue in which it began. Primary bone cancer is far less common than cancer that spreads to the bones.

Are there different types of primary bone cancer?

Yes. Cancer can begin in any type of bone tissue. Bones are made up of osteoid (hard or compact), cartilaginous (tough, flexible), and fibrous (threadlike) tissue, as well as elements of bone marrow (soft, spongy tissue in the center of most bones).

Common types of primary bone cancer include the following:

- Osteosarcoma, which arises from osteoid tissue in the bone. This tumor occurs most often in the knee and upper arm.

- Chondrosarcoma, which begins in cartilaginous tissue. Cartilage pads the ends of bones and lines the joints. Chondrosarcoma occurs most often in the pelvis (located between the hip bones), upper leg, and shoulder. Sometimes a chondrosarcoma contains cancerous bone cells. In that case, doctors classify the tumor as an osteosarcoma.

- The Ewing Sarcoma Family of Tumors (ESFTs), which usually occur in bone but may also arise in soft tissue (muscle, fat, fibrous tissue, blood vessels, or other supporting tissue). Scientists think that ESFTs arise from elements of primitive nerve tissue in the bone or soft tissue. ESFTs occur most commonly along the backbone and pelvis and in the legs and arms.

Other types of cancer that arise in soft tissue are called soft tissue sarcomas. They are not bone cancer and are not described in this resource.

What are the possible causes of bone cancer?

Although bone cancer does not have a clearly defined cause, researchers have identified several factors that increase the likelihood of developing these tumors. Osteosarcoma occurs more frequently in people who have had high-dose external radiation therapy or treatment with certain anticancer drugs; children seem to be particularly susceptible. A small number of bone cancers are due to heredity. For example, children who have had hereditary retinoblastoma (an uncommon cancer of the eye) are at a higher risk of developing osteosarcoma, particularly if they are treated with radiation. Additionally, people who have hereditary defects of bones and people with metal implants, which doctors sometimes use to repair fractures, are more likely to develop osteosarcoma. Ewing sarcoma is not strongly associated with any heredity cancer syndromes, congenital childhood diseases, or previous radiation exposure.

How often does bone cancer occur?

Primary bone cancer is rare. It accounts for much less than 1 percent of all cancers. About 2,300 new cases of primary bone cancer are diagnosed in the United States each year. Different types of bone cancer are more likely to occur in certain populations:

- Osteosarcoma occurs most commonly between ages 10 and 19. However, people over age 40 who have other conditions, such as Paget disease (a benign condition characterized by abnormal development of new bone cells), are at increased risk of developing this cancer.
- Chondrosarcoma occurs mainly in older adults (over age 40). The risk increases with advancing age. This disease rarely occurs in children and adolescents.
- ESFTs occur most often in children and adolescents under 19 years of age. Boys are

affected more often than girls. These tumors are extremely rare in African American children.

What are the symptoms of bone cancer?

Pain is the most common symptom of bone cancer, but not all bone cancers cause pain. Persistent or unusual pain or swelling in or near a bone can be caused by cancer or by other conditions. It is important to see a doctor to determine the cause.

How is bone cancer diagnosed?

To help diagnose bone cancer, the doctor asks about the patient's personal and family medical history. The doctor also performs a physical examination and may order laboratory and other diagnostic tests. These tests may include the following:

- X-rays, which can show the location, size, and shape of a bone tumor. If x-rays suggest that an abnormal area may be cancer, the doctor is likely to recommend special imaging tests. Even if x-rays suggest that an abnormal area is benign, the doctor may want to do further tests, especially if the patient is experiencing unusual or persistent pain.

- A bone scan, which is a test in which a small amount of radioactive material is injected into a blood vessel and travels through the bloodstream; it then collects in the bones and is detected by a scanner.
- A computed tomography (CT or CAT) scan, which is a series of detailed pictures of areas inside the body, taken from different angles, that are created by a computer linked to an x-ray machine.
- A magnetic resonance imaging (MRI) procedure, which uses a powerful magnet linked to a computer to create detailed pictures of areas inside the body without using x-rays.
- A positron emission tomography (PET) scan, in which a small amount of radioactive glucose (sugar) is injected into a vein, and a scanner is used to make detailed, computerized pictures of areas inside the body where the glucose is used. Because cancer cells often use more

glucose than normal cells, the pictures can be used to find cancer cells in the body.

  o An angiogram, which is an x-ray of blood vessels.

- Biopsy (removal of a tissue sample from the bone tumor) to determine whether cancer is present. The surgeon may perform a needle biopsy or an incisional biopsy. During a needle biopsy, the surgeon makes a small hole in the bone and removes a sample of tissue from the tumor with a needle-like instrument. In an incisional biopsy, the surgeon cuts into the tumor and removes a sample of tissue. Biopsies are best done by an orthopedic oncologist (a doctor experienced in the treatment of bone cancer). A pathologist (a doctor who identifies disease by studying cells and tissues under a microscope) examines the tissue to determine whether it is cancerous.

- Blood tests to determine the level of an enzyme called alkaline phosphatase. A large amount of this enzyme is present in the blood when the cells that form bone tissue are very active—when children are growing, when a broken bone is mending, or when a disease or tumor causes production of abnormal bone tissue. Because high levels of alkaline phosphatase are normal in growing children and adolescents, this test is not a completely reliable indicator of bone cancer.

What are the treatment options for bone cancer?

Treatment options depend on the type, size, location, and stage of the cancer, as well as the person's age and general health. Treatment options for bone cancer include surgery, chemotherapy, radiation therapy, and cryosurgery.

- Surgery is the usual treatment for bone cancer. The surgeon removes the entire tumor with negative margins (no cancer cells are found at the edge or border of the tissue removed during surgery). The surgeon may also use special surgical techniques to minimize the amount of healthy tissue removed with the tumor. Dramatic improvements in surgical techniques and preoperative tumor treatment have made it possible for most patients with bone cancer in an arm or leg to avoid radical surgical procedures (removal of the entire limb). However, most patients who undergo limb-sparing surgery need reconstructive surgery to maximize limb function.

- Chemotherapy is the use of anticancer drugs to kill cancer cells. Patients who have bone cancer usually receive a combination of anticancer drugs. However, chemotherapy is not currently used to treat chondrosarcoma.
- Radiation therapy, also called radiotherapy, involves the use of high-energy x-rays to kill cancer cells. This treatment may be used in combination with surgery. It is often used to treat chondrosarcoma, which cannot be treated with chemotherapy, as well as ESFTs. It may also be used for patients who refuse surgery.
- Cryosurgery is the use of liquid nitrogen to freeze and kill cancer cells. This technique can sometimes be used instead of conventional surgery to destroy the tumor.

Is follow-up treatment necessary? What does it involve?

Yes. Bone cancer sometimes metastasizes, particularly to the lungs, or can recur (come back), either at the same location or in other bones in the body. People who have had bone cancer should see their doctor regularly and should report any unusual symptoms right away. Follow-up varies for different types and stages of bone cancer. Generally, patients are checked frequently by their doctor and have regular blood tests and x-rays. People who have had bone cancer, particularly children and adolescents, have an increased likelihood of developing another type of cancer, such as leukemia, later in life. Regular follow-up care ensures that changes in health are discussed and that problems are treated as soon as possible.

Are clinical trials available for people with bone cancer?

Yes. Participation in clinical trials is an important treatment option for many people with bone cancer. To develop new treatments and better ways to use current treatments, NCI, a part of the National Institutes of Health, is sponsoring clinical trials in many hospitals and cancer centers around the country. Clinical trials are a critical step in the development of new methods of treatment. Before any new treatment can be recommended for general use, doctors conduct clinical trials to find out whether the treatment is safe for patients and effective against the disease.

People interested in taking part in a clinical trial should talk with their doctor. Information about clinical trials is available

from NCI's Cancer Information Service (CIS) at 1–800–4–
CANCER (1–800–422–6237).

Chapter 3: Childhood Cancers

- Leukemias and cancers of the brain and central nervous system account for more than half of childhood cancers.
- The causes of childhood cancers are largely unknown.
- The National Cancer Institute is funding studies examining the causes of and the most effective treatments for childhood cancers.

What are the most common types of childhood cancer?

Among the 12 major types of childhood cancers, leukemias (blood cell cancers) and cancers of the brain and central nervous system account for more than half of the new cases. About one-third of childhood cancers are leukemias. The most common type of leukemia in children is acute lymphoblastic leukemia. The most common solid tumors are brain tumors (e.g., gliomas and medulloblastomas), with other solid tumors (e.g., neuroblastomas, Wilms tumors, and sarcomas such as rhabdomyosarcoma and osteosarcoma) being less common.

How many children are diagnosed with cancer in the United States annually?

In the United States in 2007, approximately 10,400 children under age 15 were diagnosed with cancer and about 1,545 children will die from the disease. Although this makes cancer the leading cause of death by disease among U.S. children 1 to 14 years of age, cancer is still relatively rare in this age group. On average, 1 to 2 children develop the disease each year for every 10,000 children in the United States.

How have childhood cancer incidence and survival rates changed over the years?

Over the past 20 years, there has been some increase in the incidence of children diagnosed with all forms of invasive cancer, from 11.5 cases per 100,000 children in 1975 to 14.8 per 100,000 children in 2004. During this same time, however, death rates declined dramatically and 5-year survival rates increased for most childhood cancers. For example, the 5-year survival rates for all childhood cancers combined increased from 58.1 percent in 1975–77 to 79.6 percent in 1996–2003. This improvement in survival rates is due to significant advances in treatment, resulting in a cure or long-term remission for a substantial proportion of children with cancer.

Long-term trends in incidence for leukemias and brain tumors, the most common childhood cancers, show patterns that are somewhat different from the others. Incidence of childhood leukemias appeared to rise in the early 1980s, with rates increasing from 3.3 cases per 100,000 in 1975 to 4.6 cases per 100,000 in 1985. Rates in the succeeding years have shown no consistent upward or downward trend and have ranged from 3.7 to 4.9 cases per 100,000.

For childhood brain tumors, the overall incidence rose from 1975 through 2004, from 2.3 to 3.2 cases per 100,000, with the greatest increase occurring from 1983 through 1986. An article in the September 2, 1998, issue of the Journal of the National Cancer Institute suggests that the rise in incidence from 1983 through 1986 may not have represented a true increase in the number of cases, but may have reflected new forms of imaging equipment (magnetic resonance imaging or MRI) that enabled visualization of brain tumors that could not be easily visualized with older equipment. Other important developments during this time period included the changing classification of brain tumors, which resulted in tumors previously designated as "benign" being reclassified as "malignant," and improvements in neurosurgical techniques for biopsying brain tumors. Regardless of the explanation for the increase in incidence that occurred from 1983 to 1986, childhood brain tumor incidence has been essentially stable since the mid-1980s.

What are the known or suspected causes of childhood cancer?

The causes of childhood cancers are largely unknown. A few conditions, such as Down syndrome, other specific chromosomal and genetic abnormalities, and ionizing radiation exposures, explain a small percentage of cases. Environmental causes of childhood cancer have long been suspected by many scientists but have been difficult to pin down, partly because cancer in children is rare and because it is difficult to identify past exposure levels in children, particularly during potentially important periods such as pregnancy or even prior to conception. In addition, each of the distinctive types of childhood cancers develops differently—with a potentially wide variety of causes and a unique clinical course in terms of age, race, gender, and many other factors.

A number of studies are examining suspected or possible risk factors for childhood cancers, including early-life exposures to infectious agents; parental, fetal, or childhood exposures to environmental toxins such as pesticides, solvents, or other household chemicals; parental occupational exposures to radiation or chemicals; parental medical conditions during pregnancy or before conception; maternal diet during pregnancy; early postnatal feeding patterns and diet; and maternal reproductive history. Researchers are also studying the risks associated with maternal exposures to oral contraceptives, fertility drugs, and other medications; familial and genetic susceptibility; and risk associated with exposure to the human immunodeficiency virus (HIV).

What have studies shown about the possible causes of childhood cancer?

For several decades, the National Cancer Institute, a part of the National Institutes of Health (NIH), has supported national and international collaborations devoted to studying the causes of cancer in children. Key findings from this research include the following:

- High levels of ionizing radiation from accidents or from radiotherapy have been linked with increased risk of some childhood cancers.
- Children with cancer treated with chemotherapy and/or radiation therapy may be at increased risk

for developing a second primary cancer. For example, certain types of chemotherapy, including alkylating agents or topoisomerase II inhibitors (e.g., epipodophyllotoxins), can cause an increased risk of leukemia.

- Recent research has shown that children with AIDS (acquired immunodeficiency syndrome), like adults with AIDS, have an increased risk of developing certain cancers, predominantly non-Hodgkin lymphoma and Kaposi sarcoma. These children also have an additional risk of developing leiomyosarcoma (a type of muscle cancer).

- Certain genetic syndromes (e.g., Li-Fraumeni syndrome, neurofibromatosis, and Gorlin syndrome) have been linked to an increased risk of specific childhood cancers.

- Children with Down syndrome have an increased risk of developing leukemia.

- Low levels of radiation exposure from indoor radon have not been significantly associated with childhood leukemias.

- Ultrasound use during pregnancy has not been linked with childhood cancer in numerous large studies.
- Residential magnetic field exposure from power lines has not been significantly associated with childhood leukemias.
- Pesticides have been suspected to be involved in the development of certain forms of childhood cancer based on interview data. However, interview results have been inconsistent and have not yet been validated by physical evidence of pesticides in the child's body or environment.
- No consistent findings have been observed linking specific occupational exposures of parents to the development of childhood cancers.
- Several studies have found no link between maternal cigarette smoking before pregnancy and childhood cancers, but increased risks have been related to the father's smoking habits in studies in the United Kingdom and China.
- Little evidence has been found to link specific viruses or other infectious agents to the development of most types of childhood cancers, though investigators worldwide are exploring the

role of exposures of very young children to some common infectious agents that may protect children from, or put them at risk for, developing certain leukemias.

Chapter 4: Head and Neck Cancers

- Most head and neck cancers begin in the squamous cells that line the moist surfaces inside the head and neck.
- Tobacco use, alcohol use, and human papillomavirus infection are important risk factors for head and neck cancers.
- Typical symptoms of head and neck cancers include a lump or sore (for example, in the mouth) that does not heal, a sore throat that does not go away, difficulty swallowing, and a change or hoarseness in the voice.
- Rehabilitation and regular follow-up care are important parts of treatment for patients with head and neck cancers.

What are cancers of the head and neck?

Cancers that are known collectively as head and neck cancers usually begin in the squamous cells that line the moist, mucosal surfaces inside the head and neck (for example, inside the mouth, the nose, and the throat). These squamous cell cancers are often referred to as squamous cell carcinomas of the head and neck. Head and neck cancers can also begin in the salivary glands, but salivary gland cancers are relatively uncommon. Salivary glands contain many different types of cells that can become cancerous, so there are many different types of salivary gland cancer.

Cancers of the head and neck are further categorized by the area of the head or neck in which they begin.

- *Oral cavity*: Includes the lips, the front two-thirds of the tongue, the gums, the lining inside the cheeks and lips, the floor (bottom) of the mouth under the tongue, the hard palate (bony top of the mouth), and the small area of the gum behind the wisdom teeth.

- *Pharynx*: The pharynx (throat) is a hollow tube about 5 inches long that starts behind the nose and leads to the esophagus. It has three parts: the nasopharynx (the upper part of the pharynx, behind the nose); the oropharynx (the middle part of the pharynx, including the soft palate [the back of the mouth], the base of the tongue, and the tonsils); the hypopharynx (the lower part of the pharynx).

- *Larynx*: The larynx, also called the voicebox, is a short passageway formed by cartilage just below the pharynx in the neck. The larynx contains the vocal cords. It also has a small piece of tissue, called the epiglottis, which moves to cover the larynx to prevent food from entering the air passages.

- *Paranasal sinuses and nasal cavity*: The paranasal sinuses are small hollow spaces in the bones of the head surrounding the nose. The nasal cavity is the hollow space inside the nose.
- *Salivary glands*: The major salivary glands are in the floor of the mouth and near the jawbone. The salivary glands produce saliva.

Cancers of the brain, the eye, the esophagus, and the thyroid gland, as well as those of the scalp, skin, muscles, and bones of the head and neck, are not usually classified as head and neck cancers.

Sometimes, cancerous squamous cells can be found in the lymph nodes of the upper neck when there is no evidence of cancer in other parts of the head and neck. When this happens, the cancer is called metastatic squamous neck cancer with unknown (occult) primary.

What causes cancers of the head and neck?

Alcohol and tobacco use (including smokeless tobacco, sometimes called "chewing tobacco" or "snuff") are the two most important risk factors for head and neck cancers, especially cancers of the oral cavity, oropharynx, hypopharynx, and larynx. At least 75 percent of head and neck cancers are caused by tobacco and alcohol use. People who use both tobacco and alcohol are at greater risk of developing these cancers than people who use either tobacco or alcohol alone. Tobacco and alcohol use are not risk factors for salivary gland cancers.

Infection with cancer-causing types of human papillomavirus (HPV), especially HPV-16, is a risk factor for some types of head and neck cancers, particularly oropharyngeal cancers that involve the tonsils or the base of the tongue. In the United States, the incidence of oropharyngeal cancers caused by HPV infection is increasing, while the incidence of oropharyngeal cancers related to other causes is falling. Other risk factors for cancers of the head and neck include the following:

- *Paan (betel quid).* Immigrants from Southeast Asia who use paan (betel quid) in the mouth should be aware that this habit has been strongly associated with an increased risk of oral cancer.

- *Maté.* Consumption of maté, a tea-like beverage habitually consumed by South Americans, has been associated with an increased risk of cancers of the mouth, throat, esophagus, and larynx.
- *Preserved or salted foods.* Consumption of certain preserved or salted foods during childhood is a risk factor for nasopharyngeal cancer.
- *Oral health.* Poor oral hygiene and missing teeth may be weak risk factors for cancers of the oral cavity. Use of mouthwash that has a high alcohol content is a possible, but not proven, risk factor for cancers of the oral cavity.
- *Occupational exposure.* Occupational exposure to wood dust is a risk factor for nasopharyngeal cancer. Certain industrial exposures, including exposures to asbestos and synthetic fibers, have been associated with cancer of the larynx, but the increase in risk remains controversial. People working in certain jobs in the construction, metal, textile, ceramic, logging, and food industries may have an increased risk of cancer of the larynx. Industrial exposure to wood or nickel dust or formaldehyde is a risk factor for cancers of the paranasal sinuses and nasal cavity.

- *Radiation exposure.* Radiation to the head and neck, for noncancerous conditions or cancer, is a risk factor for cancer of the salivary glands.
- *Epstein-Barr virus infection.* Infection with the Epstein-Barr virus is a risk factor for nasopharyngeal cancer and cancer of the salivary glands.
- *Ancestry.* Asian ancestry, particularly Chinese ancestry, is a risk factor for nasopharyngeal cancer.

What are the symptoms of head and neck cancers?

The symptoms of head and neck cancers may include a lump or a sore that does not heal, a sore throat that does not go away, difficulty in swallowing, and a change or hoarseness in the voice. These symptoms may also be caused by other, less serious conditions. It is important to check with a doctor or dentist about any of these symptoms. Symptoms that may affect specific areas of the head and neck include the following:

- *Oral cavity.* A white or red patch on the gums, the tongue, or the lining of the mouth; a swelling of the jaw that causes dentures to fit poorly or become uncomfortable; and unusual bleeding or pain in the mouth.

- *Pharynx.* Trouble breathing or speaking; pain when swallowing; pain in the neck or the throat that does not go away; frequent headaches, pain, or ringing in the ears; or trouble hearing.
- *Larynx.* Pain when swallowing or ear pain.
- *Paranasal sinuses and nasal cavity.* Sinuses that are blocked and do not clear; chronic sinus infections that do not respond to treatment with antibiotics; bleeding through the nose; frequent headaches, swelling or other trouble with the eyes; pain in the upper teeth; or problems with dentures.
- *Salivary glands.* Swelling under the chin or around the jawbone, numbness or paralysis of the muscles in the face, or pain in the face, the chin, or the neck that does not go away.

How common are head and neck cancers?

Head and neck cancers account for approximately 3 percent of all cancers in the United States. These cancers are nearly twice as common among men as they are among women.

Head and neck cancers are also diagnosed more often among people over age 50 than they are among younger people. Researchers estimated that more than 52,000 men and women in this country would be diagnosed with head and neck cancers in 2012.

How can I reduce my risk of developing head and neck cancers?

People who are at risk of head and neck cancers—particularly those who use tobacco—should talk with their doctor about ways that they may be able to reduce their risk. They should also discuss with their doctor how often to have checkups. In addition, ongoing clinical trials are testing the effectiveness of various medications in preventing head and neck cancers in people who have a high risk of developing these diseases.

Avoiding oral HPV infection may reduce the risk of HPV-associated head and neck cancers. However, it is not yet known whether the Food and Drug Administration-approved HPV vaccines Gardasil® and Cervarix® prevent HPV infection of the oral cavity, and neither vaccine has yet been approved for the prevention of oropharyngeal cancer.

How are head and neck cancers diagnosed?

To find the cause of the signs or symptoms of a problem in the head and neck area, a doctor evaluates a person's medical history, performs a physical examination, and orders diagnostic tests. The exams and tests may vary depending on the symptoms. Examination of a sample of tissue under a microscope is always necessary to confirm a diagnosis of cancer.

If the diagnosis is cancer, the doctor will want to learn the stage (or extent) of disease. Staging is a careful attempt to find out whether the cancer has spread and, if so, to which parts of the body. Staging may involve an examination under anesthesia (in an operating room), x-rays and other imaging procedures, and laboratory tests. Knowing the stage of the disease helps the doctor plan treatment.

How are head and neck cancers treated?

The treatment plan for an individual patient depends on a number of factors, including the exact location of the tumor, the stage of the cancer, and the person's age and general health. Treatment for head and neck cancer can include surgery, radiation therapy, chemotherapy, targeted therapy, or a combination of treatments.

People who are diagnosed with HPV-positive oropharyngeal cancer may be treated differently than people with oropharyngeal cancers that are HPV-negative. Recent research has shown that patients with HPV-positive oropharyngeal tumors have a better prognosis and may do just as well on less intense treatment. An ongoing clinical trial is investigating this question.

Types of head and neck cancer are the following:

- Hypopharyngeal Cancer
- Laryngeal Cancer
- Lip and Oral Cavity Cancer
- Metastatic Squamous Neck Cancer with Occult Primary
- Nasopharyngeal Cancer
- Oropharyngeal Cancer
- Paranasal Sinus and Nasal Cavity Cancer
- Salivary Gland Cancer

Each type of head and neck cancer has specific treatment plans. The patient and the doctor should consider treatment options carefully. They should discuss each type of treatment and how it might change the way the patient looks, talks, eats, or breathes.

What are the side effects of treatment?

Surgery for head and neck cancers often changes the patient's ability to chew, swallow, or talk. The patient may look different after surgery, and the face and neck may be swollen. The swelling usually goes away within a few weeks. However, if lymph nodes are removed, the flow of lymph in the area where they were removed may be slower and lymph could collect in the tissues, causing additional swelling; this swelling may last for a long time.

After a laryngectomy (surgery to remove the larynx) or other surgery in the neck, parts of the neck and throat may feel numb because nerves have been cut. If lymph nodes in the neck were removed, the shoulder and neck may become weak and stiff.

Patients who receive radiation to the head and neck may experience redness, irritation, and sores in the mouth; a dry mouth or thickened saliva; difficulty in swallowing; changes in taste; or nausea. Other problems that may occur during treatment are loss of taste, which may decrease appetite and affect nutrition, and earaches (caused by the hardening of ear wax). Patients may also notice some swelling or drooping of the skin under the chin and changes in the texture of the skin. The jaw may feel stiff, and patients may not be able to open their mouth as wide as before treatment.

Patients should report any side effects to their doctor or nurse, and discuss how to deal with them.

Where can I find more information about clinical trials for patients with head and neck cancers?

Clinical trials are research studies conducted with people who volunteer to take part. Participation in clinical trials is an option for many patients with head and neck cancer. A list of clinical trials to treat head and neck cancers can be found at www.cancer.gov/clinicaltrials/search/results?protocolsearchid=11707657&vers=1

People interested in taking part in a clinical trial should talk with their doctor.

The National Cancer Institute provides information about specific clinical trials for people who have head and neck cancers. Questions about these trials can be answered by NCI's Cancer Information Service at 1–800–4–CANCER.

What rehabilitation or support options are available for patients with head and neck cancers?

The goal of treatment for head and neck cancers is to control the disease, but doctors are also concerned about preserving the function of the affected areas as much as they can and helping the patient return to normal activities as soon as possible after treatment. Rehabilitation is a very important part of this process. The goals of rehabilitation depend on the extent of the disease and the treatment that a patient has received.

Depending on the location of the cancer and the type of treatment, rehabilitation may include physical therapy, dietary counseling, speech therapy, and/or learning how to care for a stoma. A stoma is an opening into the windpipe through which a patient breathes after a laryngectomy, which is surgery to remove the larynx.

Sometimes, especially with cancer of the oral cavity, a patient may need reconstructive and plastic surgery to rebuild bones or tissues. However, reconstructive surgery may not always be possible because of damage to the remaining tissue from the original surgery or from radiation therapy. If reconstructive surgery is not possible, a prosthodontist may be able to make a prosthesis (an artificial dental and/or facial part) to restore satisfactory swallowing, speech, and appearance. Patients will receive special training on how to use the device.

Patients who have trouble speaking after treatment may need speech therapy. Often, a speech-language pathologist will visit the patient in the hospital to plan therapy and teach speech exercises or alternative methods of speaking. Speech therapy usually continues after the patient returns home.

Eating may be difficult after treatment for head and neck cancer. Some patients receive nutrients directly into a vein after surgery or need a feeding tube until they can eat on their own. A feeding tube is a flexible plastic tube that is passed into the stomach through the nose or an incision in the abdomen. A nurse or speech-language pathologist can help patients learn how to swallow again after surgery.

Is follow-up care necessary? What does it involve?

Regular follow-up care is very important after treatment for head and neck cancer to make sure that the cancer has not returned, or that a second primary (new) cancer has not developed. Depending on the type of cancer, medical checkups could include exams of the stoma, if one has been created, and of the mouth, neck, and throat. Regular dental exams may also be necessary.

From time to time, the doctor may perform a complete physical exam, blood tests, x-rays, and computed tomography (CT), positron emission tomography (PET), or magnetic resonance imaging (MRI) scans. The doctor may monitor thyroid and pituitary gland function, especially if the head or neck was treated with radiation. Also, the doctor is likely to counsel patients to stop smoking. Research has shown that continued smoking by a patient with head and neck cancer may reduce the effectiveness of treatment and increase the chance of a second primary cancer.

How can people who have had head and neck cancers reduce their risk of developing a second primary (new) cancer?

People who have been treated for head and neck cancers have an increased chance of developing a new cancer, usually in the head, neck, esophagus, or lungs. The chance of a second primary cancer varies depending on the site of the original cancer, but it is higher for people who use tobacco and drink alcohol.

Especially because patients who smoke have a higher risk of a second primary cancer, doctors encourage patients who use tobacco to quit. The federal government's main resource to help people quit using tobacco is BeTobaccoFree.gov. The toll-free number 1–800–QUIT–NOW (1–800–784–8669) also serves as a single point of access to state-based telephone quitlines.

Chapter 5: Inflammatory Breast Cancer

- Inflammatory breast cancer is a rare and very aggressive disease with symptoms that include redness, swelling, tenderness, and warmth in the breast.
- Treatment for inflammatory breast cancer is usually more aggressive than treatment for most other types of breast cancer.
- People with inflammatory breast cancer are encouraged to enroll in clinical trials that are testing new treatments.

What is inflammatory breast cancer?

Inflammatory breast cancer is a rare and very aggressive disease in which cancer cells block lymph vessels in the skin of the breast. This type of breast cancer is called "inflammatory" because the breast often looks swollen and red, or "inflamed."

Inflammatory breast cancer accounts for 1 to 5 percent of all breast cancers diagnosed in the United States. Most inflammatory breast cancers are invasive ductal carcinomas, which means they developed from cells that line the milk ducts of the breast and then spread beyond the ducts.

Inflammatory breast cancer progresses rapidly, often in a matter of weeks or months. Inflammatory breast cancer is either stage III or IV at diagnosis, depending on whether cancer cells have spread only to nearby lymph nodes or to other tissues as well.

Additional features of inflammatory breast cancer include the following:

- Compared with other types of breast cancer, inflammatory breast cancer tends to be diagnosed at younger ages (median age of 57 years, compared with a median age of 62 years for other types of breast cancer).

- It is more common and diagnosed at younger ages in African American women than in white women. The median age at diagnosis in African American women is 54 years, compared with a median age of 58 years in white women.

- Inflammatory breast tumors are frequently hormone receptor negative, which means that hormone therapies, such as tamoxifen, that interfere with the growth of cancer cells fueled by estrogen may not be effective against these tumors.

- Inflammatory breast cancer is more common in obese women than in women of normal weight.

Like other types of breast cancer, inflammatory breast cancer can occur in men, but usually at an older age (median age at diagnosis of 66.5 years) than in women.

What are the symptoms of inflammatory breast cancer?

Symptoms of inflammatory breast cancer include swelling (edema) and redness (erythema) that affect a third or more of the breast. The skin of the breast may also appear pink, reddish purple, or bruised. In addition, the skin may have ridges or appear pitted, like the skin of an orange (called peau d'orange). These symptoms are caused by the buildup of fluid (lymph) in the skin of the breast. This fluid buildup occurs because cancer cells have blocked lymph vessels in the skin, preventing the normal flow of lymph through the tissue. Sometimes, the breast may contain a solid tumor that can be felt during a physical exam, but, more often, a tumor cannot be felt.

Other symptoms of inflammatory breast cancer include a rapid increase in breast size; sensations of heaviness, burning, or tenderness in the breast; or a nipple that is inverted (facing inward). Swollen lymph nodes may also be present under the arm, near the collarbone, or in both places. It is important to note that these symptoms may also be signs of other diseases or conditions, such as an infection, injury, or another type of breast cancer that is locally advanced. For this reason, women with inflammatory breast cancer often have a delayed diagnosis of their disease.

How is inflammatory breast cancer diagnosed?

Inflammatory breast cancer can be difficult to diagnose. Often, there is no lump that can be felt during a physical exam or seen in a screening mammogram. In addition, most women diagnosed with inflammatory breast cancer have non-fatty (dense) breast tissue, which makes cancer detection in a screening mammogram more difficult. Also, because inflammatory breast cancer is so aggressive, it can arise between scheduled screening mammograms and progress quickly. The symptoms of inflammatory breast cancer may be mistaken for those of mastitis, which is an infection of the breast, or another form of locally advanced breast cancer. To help prevent delays in diagnosis and in choosing the best course of treatment, an international panel of experts published guidelines on how doctors can diagnose and stage inflammatory breast cancer correctly. Their recommendations are summarized below.

Minimum criteria for a diagnosis of inflammatory breast cancer include the following:

- A rapid onset of erythema (redness), edema (swelling), and a peau d'orange appearance and/or abnormal breast warmth, with or without a lump that can be felt.
- The above-mentioned symptoms have been present for less than 6 months.
- The erythema covers at least a third of the breast.
- Initial biopsy samples from the affected breast show invasive carcinoma.

Further examination of tissue from the affected breast should include testing to see if the cancer cells have hormone receptors (estrogen and progesterone receptors) or a mutation that causes them to make greater than normal amounts of the HER2 protein (HER2-positive breast cancer).

Imaging and staging tests should include the following:

- A diagnostic mammogram and an ultrasound of the breast and regional (nearby) lymph nodes.
- A PET scan or a CT scan and a bone scan to see if the cancer has spread to other parts of the body.

Proper diagnosis and staging of cancer helps doctors develop the best treatment plan and estimate the likely outcome of the disease, including the chances for recurrence and survival.

How is inflammatory breast cancer treated?

Inflammatory breast cancer is treated first with systemic chemotherapy to help shrink the tumor, then with surgery to remove the tumor, followed by radiation therapy. This approach to treatment is called a multimodal approach. Studies have found that women with inflammatory breast cancer who are treated with a multi-modal approach have better responses to therapy and longer survival. Treatments used in a multimodal approach may include those described below.

- Neoadjuvant chemotherapy: This type of chemotherapy is given before surgery and usually includes both anthracycline and taxane drugs. At least six cycles of neoadjuvant chemotherapy given over the course of 4 to 6 months before attempting to remove the tumor has been recommended, unless the disease continues to progress during this time and doctors decide that surgery should not be delayed.

- Targeted therapy: This type of treatment may be used if a woman's biopsy samples show that her cancer cells have a tumor marker that can be targeted with specific drugs. For example, inflammatory breast cancers often produce greater than normal amounts of the HER2 protein, which means they may respond positively to drugs, such as trastuzumab (Herceptin), that target this protein. Anti-HER2 therapy can be given as part of neoadjuvant therapy and after surgery (adjuvant therapy). Studies have shown that women with inflammatory breast cancer who received trastuzumab in addition to chemotherapy have better responses to treatment and better survival.

- Hormone therapy: If a woman's biopsy samples show that her cancer cells contain hormone receptors, hormone therapy is another treatment option. For example, breast cancer cells that have estrogen receptors depend on the female hormone estrogen to promote their growth. Drugs such as tamoxifen, which prevent estrogen from binding to its receptor, and aromatase inhibitors such as letrozole, which block the body's ability to make estrogen, can cause estrogen-dependent cancer cells to stop growing and die.

- Surgery: The standard surgery for inflammatory breast cancer is a modified radical mastectomy. This surgery involves removal of the entire affected breast and most or all of the lymph nodes under the adjacent arm. Often, the lining over the underlying chest muscles is also removed, but the chest muscles are preserved. Sometimes, however, the smaller chest muscle (pectoralis minor) may be removed, too.

- Radiation therapy: Post-mastectomy radiation therapy to the chest wall under the breast that was removed is a standard part of multi-modal therapy for inflammatory breast cancer. If a woman received trastuzumab before surgery, she may continue to receive it during postoperative radiation therapy. If breast reconstruction is planned, the sequencing of the radiation therapy and reconstructive surgery may be influenced by the method of breast reconstruction used. If a breast implant is to be used, the preferred approach is to delay radiation therapy until after the reconstructive surgery. If a woman's own tissues are going to be used in breast reconstruction, it is preferable to delay reconstructive surgery until after the radiation therapy has been completed.

- Adjuvant therapy: Adjuvant systemic therapy may be given after surgery to reduce the chance of cancer recurrence. This therapy may include additional chemotherapy, antihormonal therapy, targeted therapy (such as trastuzumab), or some combination of these treatments.

- Supportive/palliative care: The goal of supportive/palliative care is to improve the quality of life of patients who have a serious or life-threatening disease, such as cancer, and to provide support to their loved ones.

What is the prognosis of patients with inflammatory breast cancer?

The prognosis, or likely outcome, for a patient diagnosed with cancer is often viewed as the chance that the cancer will be treated successfully and that the patient will recover completely. Many factors can influence a cancer patient's prognosis, including the type and location of the cancer, the stage of the disease, the patient's age and overall general health, and the extent to which the patient's disease responds to treatment.

Because inflammatory breast cancer usually develops quickly and spreads aggressively to other parts of the body, women diagnosed with this disease, in general, do not survive as long as women diagnosed with other types of breast cancer. According to statistics from the National Cancer Institute's Surveillance, Epidemiology, and End Results (SEER) program, the 5-year relative survival for women diagnosed with inflammatory breast cancer during the period from 1988 through 2001 was 34 percent, compared with a 5-year relative survival of up to 87 percent among women diagnosed with other stages of invasive breast cancers.

It is important to keep in mind, however, that these survival statistics are based on large numbers of patients and that an individual woman's prognosis could be better or worse, depending on her tumor characteristics and medical history. Women who have inflammatory breast cancer are encouraged to talk with their doctor about their prognosis, given their particular situation.

Research has shown that the following factors are associated with a better prognosis for women with inflammatory breast cancer:

- Stage of disease: Women with stage III disease have a better prognosis than women with stage IV disease. Among women who have stage III inflammatory breast cancer, about 40 percent survive at least 5 years after their diagnosis, whereas among women with stage IV inflammatory breast cancer, only about 11 percent survive for at least 5 years after their diagnosis.

- Tumor grade: Women with grade I or grade II tumors have a better prognosis than those with grade III tumors. Tumor grade is a term that describes what cancer cells look like under a microscope, with a higher grade indicating a more abnormal appearance and a more aggressive cancer that is likely to grow and spread. Among women who are diagnosed with grade I or grade II inflammatory breast cancer, 77 percent survived at least 2 years after their diagnosis, whereas among women who were diagnosed with grade III inflammatory breast cancer, 65 percent survived at least 2 years after their diagnosis.

- Ethnicity: African American women who have inflammatory breast cancer generally have a worse prognosis than women of other racial and ethnic groups. Studies have found that around 53 percent of African American women who are diagnosed with inflammatory breast cancer survive at least 2 years after diagnosis, whereas 69 percent of women from other racial and ethnic groups survive at least 2 years after diagnosis.

- Estrogen receptor status: Women with inflammatory breast whose cancer cells have estrogen receptors have a better prognosis than those whose cancer cells are estrogen receptor negative. The median survival for women with estrogen-receptor negative inflammatory breast cancer is 2 years, whereas the median survival for those with estrogen receptor-positive inflammatory breast cancer is 4 years.

- Type of treatment: Multimodal treatment of inflammatory breast cancer improves a woman's prognosis. Historically, among women who had only surgery, radiation therapy, or surgery and radiation therapy, fewer than 5 percent survived longer than 5 years. However, when women are treated with neoadjuvant chemotherapy, mastectomy, adjuvant chemotherapy, and radiation therapy, their 5-year disease-free survival ranges from 24 to 49 percent. One long-term study found that 28 percent of women with inflammatory breast cancer survived 15 years or longer after they were treated with multimodal therapy.

Ongoing research, especially at the molecular level, will increase our understanding of how inflammatory breast cancer begins and progresses. This knowledge should enable the development of new treatments and more accurate prognoses for women diagnosed with this disease. It is important, therefore, that women who are diagnosed with inflammatory breast cancer talk with their doctor about the option of participating in a clinical trial.

Chapter 6: Metastatic Cancer

- Metastatic cancer is cancer that has spread from the place where it first started to another place in the body.
- Metastatic cancer has the same name and same type of cancer cells as the original cancer.
- The most common sites of cancer metastasis are, in alphabetical order, the bone, liver, and lung.

What is metastatic cancer?

Metastatic cancer is cancer that has spread from the place where it first started to another place in the body. A tumor formed by metastatic cancer cells is called a metastatic tumor or a metastasis. The process by which cancer cells spread to other parts of the body is also called metastasis.

Metastatic cancer has the same name and the same type of cancer cells as the original, or primary, cancer. For example, breast cancer that spreads to the lung and forms a metastatic tumor is metastatic breast cancer, not lung cancer.

Under a microscope, metastatic cancer cells generally look the same as cells of the original cancer. Moreover, metastatic cancer cells and cells of the original cancer usually have some molecular features in common, such as the expression of certain proteins or the presence of specific chromosome changes.

Although some types of metastatic cancer can be cured with current treatments, most cannot. Nevertheless, treatments are available for all patients with metastatic cancer. In general, the primary goal of these treatments is to control the growth of the cancer or to relieve symptoms caused by it. In some cases, metastatic cancer treatments may help prolong life. However, most people who die of cancer die of metastatic disease.

Can any type of cancer form a metastatic tumor?

Virtually all cancers, including cancers of the blood and the lymphatic system (leukemia, multiple myeloma, and lymphoma), can form metastatic tumors. Although rare, the metastasis of blood and lymphatic system cancers to the lung, heart, central nervous system, and other tissues has been reported.

Where does cancer spread?

The most common sites of cancer metastasis are, in alphabetical order, the bone, liver, and lung. Although most cancers have the ability to spread to many different parts of the body, they usually spread to one site more often than others. The following table shows the most common sites of metastasis, excluding the lymph nodes, for several types of cancer:

Cancer Type	Main Sites of Metastasis*
Bladder	Bone, liver, lung
Breast	Bone, brain, liver, lung
Colorectal	Liver, lung, peritoneum
Kidney	Adrenal gland, bone, brain, liver, lung
Lung	Adrenal gland, bone, brain, liver, lung, other lung
Melanoma	Bone, brain, liver, lung, skin/muscle
Ovary	Liver, lung, peritoneum
Pancreas	Liver, lung, peritoneum
Prostate	Adrenal gland, blone, liver, lung
Stomach	Liver, lung, peritoneum
Thyroid	Bone, liver, lung
Uterus	Bone, liver, lung, peritoneum, vagina

*In alphabetical order. Brain includes the neural tissue of the brain (parenchyma) and the leptomeninges (the two innermost membranes—arachnoid mater and pia mater—of the three membranes known as the meninges that surround the brain and spinal cord; the space between the arachnoid mater and the pia mater contains cerebrospinal fluid). Lung includes the main part of the lung (parenchyma) as well as the pleura (the membrane that covers the lungs and lines the chest cavity).

How does cancer spread?

Cancer cell metastasis usually involves the following steps:

- *Local invasion*: Cancer cells invade nearby normal tissue.
- *Intravasation*: Cancer cells invade and move through the walls of nearby lymph vessels or blood vessels.
- *Circulation*: Cancer cells move through the lymphatic system and the bloodstream to other parts of the body.
- *Arrest and extravasation*: Cancer cells arrest, or stop moving, in small blood vessels called capillaries at a distant location. They then invade the walls of the capillaries and migrate into the surrounding tissue (extravasation).

- *Proliferation*: Cancer cells multiply at the distant location to form small tumors known as micrometastases.
- *Angiogenesis*: Micrometastases stimulate the growth of new blood vessels to obtain a blood supply. A blood supply is needed to obtain the oxygen and nutrients necessary for continued tumor growth.

Because cancers of the lymphatic system or the blood system are already present inside lymph vessels, lymph nodes, or blood vessels, not all of these steps are needed for their metastasis. Also, the lymphatic system drains into the blood system at two locations in the neck.

The ability of a cancer cell to metastasize successfully depends on its individual properties; the properties of the noncancerous cells, including immune system cells, present at the original location; and the properties of the cells it encounters in the lymphatic system or the bloodstream and at the final destination in another part of the body. Not all cancer cells, by themselves, have the ability to metastasize. In addition, the noncancerous cells at the original location may be able to block cancer cell metastasis. Furthermore, successfully reaching another location in the body does not guarantee that a metastatic tumor will form. Metastatic cancer cells can lie dormant (not grow) at a distant site for many years before they begin to grow again, if at all.

Does metastatic cancer have symptoms?

Some people with metastatic tumors do not have symptoms. Their metastases are found by x-rays or other tests.

When symptoms of metastatic cancer occur, the type and frequency of the symptoms will depend on the size and location of the metastasis. For example, cancer that spreads to the bone is likely to cause pain and can lead to bone fractures. Cancer that spreads to the brain can cause a variety of symptoms, including headaches, seizures, and unsteadiness. Shortness of breath may be a sign of lung metastasis. Abdominal swelling or jaundice (yellowing of the skin) can indicate that cancer has spread to the liver.

Sometimes a person's original cancer is discovered only after a metastatic tumor causes symptoms. For example, a man whose prostate cancer has spread to the bones in his pelvis may have lower back pain (caused by the cancer in his bones) before he experiences any symptoms from the original tumor in his prostate.

Can someone have a metastatic tumor without having a primary cancer?

No. A metastatic tumor is always caused by cancer cells from another part of the body.

In most cases, when a metastatic tumor is found first, the primary cancer can also be found. The search for the primary cancer may involve lab tests, x-rays, computed tomography (CT) scans, magnetic resonance imaging (MRI) scans, positron emission tomography (PET) scans, and other procedures.

However, in some patients, a metastatic tumor is diagnosed but the primary tumor cannot be found, despite extensive tests, because it either is too small or has completely regressed. The pathologist knows that the diagnosed tumor is a metastasis because the cells do not look like those of the organ or tissue in which the tumor was found. Doctors refer to the primary cancer as unknown or occult (hidden), and the patient is said to have cancer of unknown primary origin (CUP).

If a person who was previously treated for cancer gets diagnosed with cancer a second time, is the new cancer a new primary cancer or metastatic cancer?

The cancer may be a new primary cancer, but, in most cases, it is metastatic cancer.

What treatments are used for metastatic cancer?

Metastatic cancer may be treated with systemic therapy (chemotherapy, biological therapy, targeted therapy, hormonal therapy), local therapy (surgery, radiation therapy), or a combination of these treatments. The choice of treatment generally depends on the type of primary cancer; the size, location, and number of metastatic tumors; the patient's age and general health; and the types of treatment the patient has had in the past. In patients with CUP, it is possible to treat the disease even though the primary cancer has not been found.

Are new treatments for metastatic cancer being developed?

Yes, researchers are studying new ways to kill or stop the growth of primary cancer cells and metastatic cancer cells, including new ways to boost the strength of immune responses against tumors. In addition, researchers are trying to find ways to disrupt individual steps in the metastatic process.

Before any new treatment can be made widely available to patients, it must be studied in clinical trials (research studies) and found to be safe and effective in treating disease. The National Cancer Institute and many other organizations sponsor clinical trials that take place at hospitals, universities, medical schools, and cancer centers around the country.

Clinical trials are a critical step in improving cancer care. The results of previous clinical trials have led to progress not only in the treatment of cancer but also in the detection, diagnosis, and prevention of the disease. Patients interested in taking part in a clinical trial should talk with their doctor.

Chapter 7: Paget Disease of the Breast

- Paget disease of the breast is a rare type of cancer involving the skin of the nipple and, usually, the darker circle of skin around it, known as the areola.

- Most of the time, people with Paget disease of the breast also have one or more tumors inside the same breast.

- Paget disease of the breast may be misdiagnosed at first because its early symptoms are similar to those caused by some benign skin conditions.

- The outlook for people diagnosed with Paget disease of the breast depends on a variety of factors, including the presence or absence of invasive cancer in the affected breast and, if invasive cancer is present, whether or not it has spread to nearby lymph nodes.

What is Paget disease of the breast?

Paget disease of the breast (also known as Paget disease of the nipple and mammary Paget disease) is a rare type of cancer involving the skin of the nipple and, usually, the darker circle of skin around it, which is called the areola.

Most people with Paget disease of the breast also have one or more tumors inside the same breast. These breast tumors are either ductal carcinoma in situ or invasive breast cancer. Paget disease of the breast is named after the 19th century British doctor Sir James Paget, who, in 1874, noted a relationship between changes in the nipple and breast cancer. (Several other diseases are named after Sir James Paget, including Paget disease of bone and extramammary Paget disease, which includes Paget disease of the vulva and Paget disease of the penis. These other diseases are not related to Paget disease of the breast. This fact sheet discusses only Paget disease of the breast.)

Malignant cells known as Paget cells are a telltale sign of Paget disease of the breast. These cells are found in the epidermis (surface layer) of the skin of the nipple and the areola. Paget cells often have a large, round appearance under a microscope; they may be found as single cells or as small groups of cells within the epidermis.

Who gets Paget disease of the breast?

Paget disease of the breast occurs in both women and men, but most cases occur in women. Approximately 1 to 4 percent of all cases of breast cancer also involve Paget disease of the breast. The average age at diagnosis is 57 years, but the disease has been found in adolescents and in people in their late 80s.

What causes Paget disease of the breast?

Doctors do not fully understand what causes Paget disease of the breast. The most widely accepted theory is that cancer cells from a tumor inside the breast travel through the milk ducts to the nipple and areola. This would explain why Paget disease of the breast and tumors inside the same breast are almost always found together.

A second theory is that cells in the nipple or areola become cancerous on their own. This would explain why a few people develop Paget disease of the breast without having a tumor inside the same breast. Moreover, it may be possible for Paget disease of the breast and tumors inside the same breast to develop independently.

What are the symptoms of Paget disease of the breast?

The symptoms of Paget disease of the breast are often mistaken for those of some benign skin conditions, such as dermatitis or eczema. These symptoms may include the following:

- Itching, tingling, or redness in the nipple and/or areola
- Flaking, crusty, or thickened skin on or around the nipple
- A flattened nipple
- Discharge from the nipple that may be yellowish or bloody

Because the early symptoms of Paget disease of the breast may suggest a benign skin condition, and because the disease is rare, it may be misdiagnosed at first. People with Paget disease of the breast have often had symptoms for several months before being correctly diagnosed.

How is Paget disease of the breast diagnosed?

A nipple biopsy allows doctors to correctly diagnose Paget disease of the breast. There are several types of nipple biopsy, including the procedures described below.

- *Surface biopsy*: A glass slide or other tool is used to gently scrape cells from the surface of the skin.
- *Shave biopsy*: A razor-like tool is used to remove the top layer of skin.
- *Punch biopsy*: A circular cutting tool, called a punch, is used to remove a disk-shaped piece of tissue.

- *Wedge biopsy*: A scalpel is used to remove a small wedge of tissue.

In some cases, doctors may remove the entire nipple. A pathologist then examines the cells or tissue under a microscope to look for Paget cells.

Most people who have Paget disease of the breast also have one or more tumors inside the same breast. In addition to ordering a nipple biopsy, the doctor should perform a clinical breast exam to check for lumps or other breast changes. As many as 50 percent of people who have Paget disease of the breast have a breast lump that can be felt in a clinical breast exam. The doctor may order additional diagnostic tests, such as a diagnostic mammogram, an ultrasound exam, or a magnetic resonance imaging scan to look for possible tumors.

How is Paget disease of the breast treated?

For many years, mastectomy, with or without the removal of lymph nodes under the arm on the same side of chest (known as axillary lymph node dissection), was regarded as the standard surgery for Paget disease of the breast. This type of surgery was done because patients with Paget disease of the breast were almost always found to have one or more tumors inside the same breast. Even if only one tumor was present, that tumor could be located several centimeters away from the nipple and areola and would not be removed by surgery on the nipple and areola alone.

Studies have shown, however, that breast-conserving surgery that includes removal of the nipple and areola, followed by whole-breast radiation therapy, is a safe option for people with Paget disease of the breast who do not have a palpable lump in their breast and whose mammograms do not reveal a tumor.

People with Paget disease of the breast who have a breast tumor and are having a mastectomy should be offered sentinel lymph node biopsy to see whether the cancer has spread to the axillary lymph nodes. If cancer cells are found in the sentinel lymph node(s), more extensive axillary lymph node surgery may be needed. Depending on the stage and other features of the underlying breast tumor (for example, the presence or absence of lymph node involvement, estrogen and progesterone receptors in the tumor cells, and HER2 protein overexpression in the tumor cells), adjuvant therapy, consisting of chemotherapy and/or hormonal therapy, may also be recommended.

What is the prognosis for people with Paget disease of the breast?

The prognosis, or outlook, for people with Paget disease of the breast depends on a variety of factors, including the following:

- Whether or not a tumor is present in the affected breast
- If one or more tumors are present in the affected breast, whether those tumors are ductal carcinoma in situ or invasive breast cancer
- If invasive breast cancer is present in the affected breast, the stage of that cancer

The presence of invasive cancer in the affected breast and the spread of cancer to nearby lymph nodes are associated with reduced survival.

According to the SEER program, the 5-year relative survival for all women in the United States who were diagnosed with Paget disease of the breast between 1988 and 2001 was 82.6 percent. This compares with a 5-year relative survival of 87.1 percent for women diagnosed with any type of breast cancer. For women with both Paget disease of the breast and invasive cancer in the same breast, the 5-year relative survival declined with increasing stage of the cancer (stage I, 95.8 percent; stage II, 77.7 percent; stage III, 46.3 percent; stage IV, 14.3 percent).

What research studies are under way on Paget disease of the breast?

Randomized controlled clinical trials, which are considered the "gold standard" in cancer research, are difficult to perform for Paget disease of the breast because very few people have this disease (4, 10). However, people who have Paget disease of the breast may be eligible to enroll in clinical trials to evaluate new treatments for breast cancer in general, new ways of using existing breast cancer treatments, or strategies for preventing breast cancer recurrence.

Other MedicalCenter.com Publications

The Key Facts on Arthritis

The Key Facts on Breast Cancer

The Key Facts on Medicare

The Key Facts on Alzheimer's Disease

The Key Facts on Caring For Someone With Alzheimer's Disease

The Key Facts on Cancer Series

All Titles Can Be Found at

www.Amazon.com

www.MedicalCenter.com